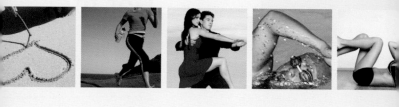

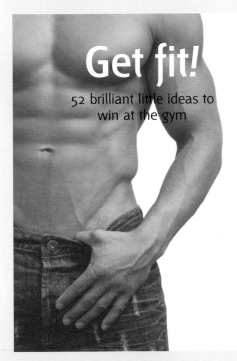

Get fit!

52 brilliant little ideas to
win at the gym

Steve Shipside

brilliantideas

CAREFUL NOW

Before beginning any exercise programme, it is advisable to obtain the approval and recommendations of your doctor. It's also advisable to visit your doctor for periodic monitoring. Know your limits and don't take risks beyond your level of experience or ability. Fix your own goals and focus on your own workout - not what other people are doing. It's your body, and it's up to you to take responsibility for your own safety and progress.

Mention of specific companies in this book does not necessarily imply endorsement by the publisher, nor does it imply that those companies endorse the book. All web addresses were checked before publication but in this fast moving world these may sometimes go out of date - so sorry for any inconvenience this may cause.

First published in 2007 by
The Infinite Ideas Company Limited
36 St Giles
Oxford, OX1 3LD
United Kingdom
www.infideas.com

A CIP catalogue record for this book is available from the British Library

ISBN 978-1-905940-19-6

Designed and typeset by Baseline Arts Ltd, Oxford
Printed in China

Brilliant ideas

Stop sniggering. This is how to make the treadmill seem less of a, well, treadmill.

Never done a marathon and curious if you could hit that time you hanker after? Looking to improve your existing time? Here's how to know if you can do either.

Ever wondered what those oversized beach balls are doing in the gym? Here's where you find out what they're for, and why they can help create a better you.

Those over-sized beach balls can also be used for strength work. So forget the fun and games, this is where the balls get their own back.

The stepper is how you forge buns of steel, but you can also get a full fat-burning cardio and core-strength workout at the same time. Shhh... here's the secret.

Sit-ups, crunches, reverse crunches – have you ever wondered if there was another way to a strong mid-section without all the bobbing up and down? There is – time to get static.

Neglect your back and no one will see your six-pack or admire your navel piercing because you'll be hunched up like Quasimodo doing his shoelaces.

Sitting on a stationary bike flipping through a paper isn't going to cut it. Try some triathlon cyclist techniques for getting better instead of just getting bored.

Turn your cycling skills into raw power by looking at strength work.

The elliptical trainer is a relatively new kid on the gym block but its popularity means that it's a rare gym without a small posse of them.

Introduction

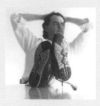

Ask yourself the following...
Are you keen to lose weight?
Want to tone up that body?
Looking for stamina and health gains?
Bored witless in the gym?

So you've got over the hurdle of hauling yourself off the couch and down to the gym. Great. You've located the lockers, you know how to use at least half the buttons on the treadmill, and you've embarked on an on–off fling with a couple of classes and a weight machine or two. But now the initial wave of enthusiasm is some way behind you, and you're not entirely sure you're getting anywhere.

Which is where this book comes in. It's written by an ordinary guy who embarked on a fitness journey that saw him go from overweight keyboard jockey to extreme triathlete. He still doesn't know what it feels like to stand on the winner's podium, but there is nothing he can't tell you about gym boredom. In order to keep training he has had to dig deep into the secrets of spicing up those gym sessions. Professional athletes, running partners, personal trainers – all the people he's ever exercised with have been frisked, pick-pocketed or brutally mugged for their ideas on how keep up the gym momentum.

Here's how to set goals, avoid burn out and measure your progress. How to use those really obscure machines that lurk menacingly in the corner of the weights room. How to banish boredom on the stationary bike and defeat the tedium of treadmill time. However unlikely it may sound, you'll find yourself having fun as you get fit.

It's intended for men and for women, for those looking to build strength as much as those hoping to burn blubber, for improvers at every level from the seriously grudging, to the wildly over-ambitious. Stick with it and you'll become an indoor triathlete, learn your marathon target time, shimmy yourself svelte and fall off objects you don't even know the name of yet.

There *is* gain without pain, you can win in the gym, and you don't have to wear legwarmers. Promise.

1. Looking the part

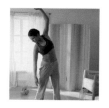

Looking the part is probably the least of your concerns, but proper gym wear can make all the difference between a good session and an afternoon in A&E.

This has nothing to do with fashion. When it comes to function the choice between good and bad gear can help you perform at your peak or wind up in hospital.

Get your footwear right. When running, the entire weight of your body crashes down on one part of your foot. We all run in different ways and one of the key differences is the way our feet take the shock. To the experts that's called *pronation*.

With a neutral footfall the first point of impact is the heel, but most of us overpronate to certain degree: our foot lands on the outside edge of the heel and rolls inwards as the weight is shifted to the ball and off again. A well-designed shoe for an overpronator

Here's an idea for you

You can get an idea of whether you're a pronator or supinator by looking at the wear on the underside of your current shoes. That will say even more to a specialist, so take your old gym shoes when you go shopping.

will cushion the outside edge of the foot. And just to make things more awkward, some people do just the opposite: *oversupinate* – they roll their feet outwards. Then some have an unusually strong heelstrike, and some strike on the ball of the foot. Each way of running requires a differently designed shoe. Go to a specialist shop where someone can see you run and suggest shoes to suit you. Wear the wrong shoes, with the wrong degree of cushioning, and you're increasing the risk of injury.

Running is just one kind of motion. The moment you indulge in martial arts, step or almost any other training you will start moving sideways, jumping and changing direction suddenly. Now you need lateral cushioning and probably ankle protection. Get a dedicated cross-trainer.

Work out and you will sweat. Sweat in cotton and your clothes will soon be sporting large, cold, damp patches, so switch to wicking fabric. Seriously good sports bras are invaluable and, finally, no jewellery – please.

2. Turning up the heat

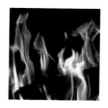

Warming up is a bit like going regularly to the dentist. We know we should, we skip it as often as we can. Here's why we should do it properly.

Warming up can mean pretty much any moderate exercise that raises the pulse gradually. Even something as simple as a couple of minutes running on the spot will suffice. The purpose of a simple warm-up is also to raise the body temperature and psychologically prepare for the session ahead. Increasing the temperature increases the elasticity of muscle, reducing the risk of injury. It also increases the metabolic rate of cells and the readiness of the nervous system. There are some basic rules.

Confusing stretching and warming up is a common mistake. Stretching muscles when cold increases the chance of hurting them and stretching on its own is unlikely to raise either your pulse or your body temperature. Try milder stretching after a bit of warm up – run gently for a few

Here's an idea for you

Getting to the gym can be made into part of your workout routine if you treat it as a warm-up. Walk there briskly and change fast, then your pulse and body temperature should still be above normal and you should be more ready for action.

minutes and then try stretching at the same time with exercises like high stepping (knees up towards chest) and high kicking (heels to bum).

If you're planning on running on the treadmill, warm up first by setting the speed. First walk comfortably, then faster, then find that point where you are striding so fast you want to break into a run and hold it there for a minute or so.

Choose a warm-up that works both upper and lower body. Even sprinters stop and do press-ups in order to increase blood flow and body temperature. And always aim to do your cardio first before going to the weights room to push metal around. Never turn up late for classes, skipping the warm-up and plunging straight into the exercises, and where there is a warm-up remember to use it as such.

3. Cool it

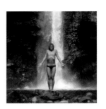

When you've done a hard session the temptation is to hit the shower/pub quickly. The success of your next session is at stake, however, if you don't take the time to cool down.

Cool-downs are mainly about getting rid of lactic acid and avoiding blood pooling in the muscles you've just worked so hard to pump full of the stuff. Coming to an abrupt halt after exercise can also cause cramps, soreness (often due to lactic acid build-up), dizziness or even abnormal strain on the heart. A good cool-down helps the body return gently to its pre-workout state with breathing and heartbeat falling to normal levels. Keeping moving also allows the blood to be pumped back from the extremities and muscles.

Probably the best and simplest cool-down is walking. A good striding motion gradually slowed down to normal pace keeps all the limbs moving rhythmically and lets the lungs catch up.

Here's an idea for you

Massage is another great way of helping your metabolism recover from the effort and trauma of your session. A good massage also helps reinforce the sense of reward and that oh-so-fab feelgood factor.

Distinguish cooling down from stretching. The best time to stretch is after you've done five to ten minutes of cool-down because your muscles will still be at their most flexible. Pretty much every gym class these days has a cool-down section at the end, and there are usually a couple of people who skip off early. It's understandable but not a good idea. Apart from anything else a proper cool-down contributes massively to the feeling of well-being and smugness after a workout and that's to be encouraged if you want your healthy habit to last.

The cool-down is also a great time to reach for that water bottle, and maybe a banana to start rehydrating and refuelling. Even if you're only in the gym because you want to lose weight, that post-exercise refuelling session is the key to ensuring your metabolism burns fat reserves rather than trying to hold on to them.

4. Take heart

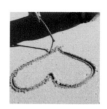

How fit are you? How do you know if you're in the fat-burning zone or working at your threshold? Let your heart show you the way.

We all exercise because we're looking for some kind of benefit – losing weight, avoiding heart attacks, living longer. But what of less obvious but often more crucial goals? Sooner or later, you'll start to wonder if it's really doing any good.

The answer is to listen to your heart, and the way to do that is to invest in a heart rate monitor. Having an accurate idea of your heart rate opens a whole new world of accuracy in training. You can now tell exactly how hard you are working, which is often different to how hard you think you are working. By seeing how long it takes for your heart to recover from bursts of exercise you have access to one of the best indicators of how fit you really are.

The first thing is to establish your maximum heart rate, and it's best

Here's an idea for you

Do your usual session and then see how long it takes your heart rate to drop to 120 (12 beats within a 10 second period if you're doing it manually). As you get fitter that time will drop, and you may find it becomes more accurate to count how long it takes to get down to 100 beats.

to follow the instructions that come with your heart monitor. Once you're at your maximum, the next step is working out the different training zones. Roughly speaking there are three main training zones: 60–75 % of max which is considered easy and often called the 'fat-burning zone', 75–85 % of max which is moderate and sometimes referred to as the 'cardio-training zone'; and 85–95 % which is normally only of interest to those going for peak performance.

The simplest monitors consist of a stop watch and will tell you what your rate is. The next step up feature alarms that can be set for zones so, for example, the monitor beeps at you if you get out of the fat-burning zone, or if you drop below a certain level of workload. Beyond that, monitors start sprouting all sorts of exciting functions.

5. Quality versus quantity

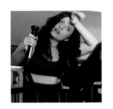

If some is good, then more must be better, right? No. Training smart can often mean training less.

What happens to many of us is that having started to go to the gym we feel better about ourselves. Being in the gym is what makes us feel good, so we may spend an extra half an hour on a machine, particularly something comfy where we can sit down. This kind of exercise isn't really training, it's more about remaining in a comfort zone. It's junk training; it lets you kid yourself you've worked out and you may let things slip elsewhere. A lot of people reward themselves for having gone to the gym, maybe with snacks afterwards or maybe more insidiously – like not taking the stairs because, well, you are going to the gym...

This doesn't mean the gym always has to be about pain, just that if you don't have a clear goal for every visit then you might be better off skipping that session.

Here's an idea for you

Muscle is denser and thus heavier than fat. If you're strength training while calorie burning you could end up in better shape but weighing more. Get yourself tested for body fat percentage either at the gym or by buying body-composition 'scales'.

Similarly if you're not feeling good enough to reach your goal, then why not take the day off and go for it next time instead? Going for quantity not quality works fine for a while, but before long you'll hit a plateau of tiredness, boredom and disappointment.

Draw up some goals, and the means of measuring them. Working out three times a week or spending five hours in the gym is what's called a *process goal* because it focuses on the process, not on the actual outcome. Start setting yourself *outcome goals* instead. Typical outcome goals tend to be along the lines of 'building bigger arms' or 'getting fitter'. A bit vague. If you want results you need to work out how to measure them and give yourself a deadline such as 'build 2 cm of muscle onto my arms by Easter'.

Now you have goals, ways to measure them and deadlines, you can go back to the gym and decide whether you're really achieving something, or just junk training.

6. I want my MP3

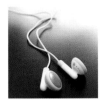

Music makes the time fly when you're performing the flywheel fandango on rowers or exercise bikes. But someone else's choice can easily put a stick in your (imaginary) spokes.

People have always liked working out to music, but they often confuse good music with good workout music. If the music is real listening music, music you want to pay attention to, then you may not be paying enough attention to the exercise you're meant to be doing. However attached you may be to a Schubert sonata or whale song you'd be best advised to leave them at home. Good workout music tends to be energetic, rousing and definitely more about beat than about lyrics.

The reason why dance and trance work so well is that they are aimed at people who are off their heads one way or another and aiming to carry on moving to the beat. You may not like to compare yourself to a nightclub full of teenagers ripped

Here's an idea for you

When you record your compilation take note of how long each song is. Next time you're on a cardio machine cover the readout with a towel, shut your eyes and keep going for a set number of songs – five, ten, whatever. Time will pass way faster than when you're watching for the moment you can stop.

23

to the gills but there are times when that mindless motion is precisely what you're aiming for.

Most gyms have canned music over speakers – which is useless for rhythm since it's half drowned out by the sound of machines. Many have radio stations or TV channels but even 'dance' channels and MTV seem to be about 50% talk. Which isn't what you want as you try to attain that trance-like out-of-body feeling that floats you ever onwards.

Bringing your own music is the answer. Don't just use that Steps CD that's lying there but make your own compilation of upbeat energy. Plenty of people make up their favourite party compilations; why do so few put the same effort into jazzing up the gym session? Putting together a selection you really want to hear will help put some spice into your next session. Guaranteed.

7. Row like Redgrave I

Strength, stamina and smoothness are the promise of the rowing machine. So why do so many users look less like Steve Redgrave and more like Mr Bean?

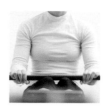

Done properly, rowing is a great calorie burner, combining weight control with strength development and a cardio workout. Beginners look at the rowing action and see two parts: the pull back and the flop forwards again. Pros, however, break the action down into four:

The catch. You're sitting on the rower and your feet are safely strapped. Slide forward so your shins are vertical, and you have the handle grasped in both hands with your wrists flat and your torso leaning slightly forwards from the hips.

The drive. The powerhouse for this is the legs and *never the arms*. Straighten those legs, pushing hard against the foot rests, and keep the arms straight for the first part of the drive. As your legs straighten

Here's an idea for you

See the lever on the flywheel that sets the difficulty level? On pretty much all rowing machines it can be set from anywhere between 1 and 10. The unsure slot the lever down to 1 and most blokes whack it up to 10. Pros tend to go for the feel that is most like a real boat, which means a level of 3 or 4. Then they concentrate on stroke rate, aiming for about 35 strokes a minute.

out and you are nearing the end of the drive, then your arms start to bend slightly and your upper body comes into play, leaning slightly backwards.

The finish. Legs straighten completely, upper body leans lightly backwards, and you pull the handle in towards your stomach just below your rib cage. At the end of the pull your elbows should be tucked in close to your body and behind your back, not sticking out sideways.

The recovery. First the arms extend forwards, then your upper body leans lightly forward, and your legs bend as you slide smoothly back towards the flywheel down by your feet. And back to the catch...

8. Row like Redgrave II

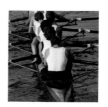

You've mastered the style and your rowing is now a symphony of power and precision. Now what? Time to step up to your own Olympic challenge.

At their peak Redgrave, Pinsent and co. didn't have to worry about getting bored or going off the boil in the gym. Us mere mortals tend to plateau – we do all right and then hit a point where training doesn't seem to bring any benefits. Interval training, however, aims to add a little spice to your gym life by mixing and matching on pace, stretching both your speed and your endurance. It can help.

First get an idea of your standard pace (and in the process give yourself a yardstick to measure progress) by rowing for 30 minutes without a break. Warm up for five minutes beforehand, and try not to go off too fast at the beginning. Pace yourself so that you have

Here's an idea for you

Instead of going for a set speed or distance, take a sample time – say ten minutes – and complete it at a fixed stroke rate, whatever you feel comfortable with. At the end of the time note the distance covered. In future, keep to the same time and stroke rate, but see if you can increase the distance.

given it all you've got by the end. Once you've got that yardstick, it's time to try a pyramid row.

This works much like pyramid sets in weightlifting. Start off gently with a warm-up for a couple of minutes, then start your pyramid. Two minutes fast rowing, followed by two minutes at a pace where you would feel easy enough to chat. Then three minutes fast, then three minutes easy, then four minutes fast, four minutes easy. That's the pyramid climbed, now for the way back down. After four minutes easy it's back to three minutes fast, then three easy, two fast, then two easy. Feeling hard? Try starting your pyramid at three minutes and going up to five, and if that doesn't get you, then try starting at four and going on to six.

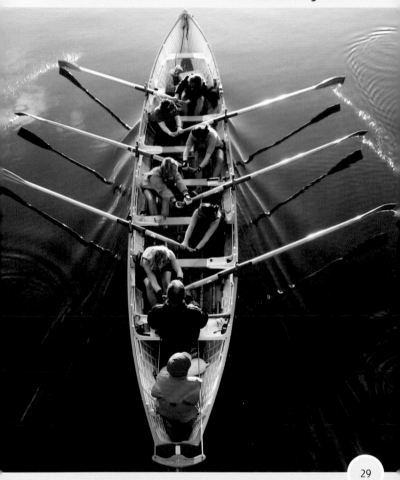

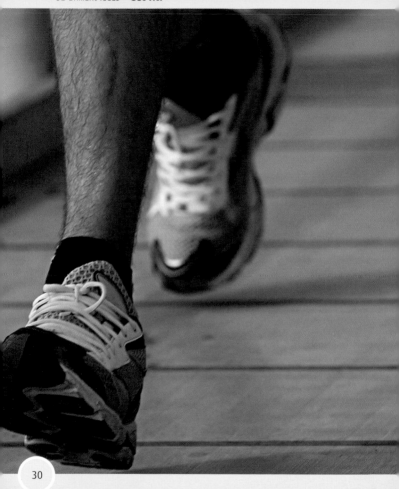

9. Run I: Fartlek

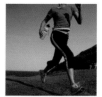

Stop sniggering. This is how to make the treadmill seem less of a, well, treadmill.

If you're already a gym regular you won't need to be told that aside from injury the biggest threat to success is boredom. Which is where fartlek comes in. It's Swedish for 'speedplay' and the idea couldn't be simpler – more varied, more interesting and more challenging running results in better runners.

The idea is to vary pace and effort, rewarding bursts of extra hard work with recovery periods at an easier rate. That's the speed part of speedplay. The play part comes in by throwing in an element of unpredictability. Fartlek runners in the open may decide to sprint to a lamppost and then take it easy to the next one as a means of varying the effort. Sessions are not measured in distance covered or speed, but in the time of the session.

Use a treadmill capable of different speeds and angles of climb. Instead of your normal run, try warming up gently for five to ten minutes then increasing the gradient dramatically for five minutes, or sprinting the

Here's an idea for you

TVs in gyms are ideal for fartlek. Try to run at above race pace for the duration of the next music video, or keep running at an incline until the next male vocalist takes to the screen.

next half a kilometre at a speed a good couple of notches up from your usual. As for the element of the unexpected, you usually have a whole gym-full of suspects who can unwittingly be roped in. Try setting a goal like sprinting for as long as the guy in the corner can bench press those car-sized weights. A good session should include a mix of alternated easy running, hard running, hill climbing, walking and absolutely flat out; what you get out depends very much on how much you put in.

Aside from the light relief of varying your routines (and never underestimate the importance of that), the great benefit of fartlek is that it prepares you for the unexpected.

10. Run II: Yasso 800s

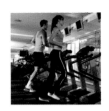

Never done a marathon and curious if you could hit that time you hanker after? Looking to improve your existing time? Here's how to know if you can do either.

There's more to running than just pegging it at the same pace all the time. By running at above normal pace for short intervals, then resting by running more slowly ('active recovery') you can train yourself to run faster for longer. Interval training for runners usually seems to involve a track, someone with a stopwatch and a complicated formula of distances and times. Yasso 800s give you the performance goals of intervals with a pretty fair idea of whether you could achieve your marathon goal. They get their name from Bart Yasso, who noticed a direct link between the time he took to run a marathon and the time he took to run a series of 800 metres (about half a mile).

The idea is simple. Say you've always felt that you had it in you to complete a marathon in four hours. Take that time, and you have your 800 m goal – only in minutes. Now do 800 m in four minutes on the

Here's an idea for you

Never seriously thought of running a marathon but can run four or five kilometres? Well go and try a couple of Yasso 800s, see what you can do, and start dreaming about whether you could go for the big one.

treadmill, then 'rest' by dropping the speed and running gently for the same number of minutes. Then you try to do another 800 m in four minutes, then rest for the same time.

The same principle seems to work whatever your speed. If you think it would take five hours to go the distance, then working on five-minute 800s should see you through. And once you've set your goal you're not going to have trouble remembering what time you're meant to run 800 m intervals in. Just one thing to remember: Bart Yasso runs outdoors, you're on a treadmill with no wind resistance. To compensate, you should up the treadmill incline to 1%.

It isn't guaranteed to be 100% accurate, because we're all different, but it should help. It can also be a reality check for the over-ambitious.

11. Balls I

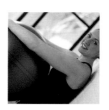

Ever wondered what those oversized beach balls are doing in the gym? Here's where you find out what they're for, and why they can help create a better you.

Swiss balls are just wonderful. They're big, they're soft – and they're the key to great stretches and core strength, which translates to a flat stomach. The first thing to know about them is that they aren't all the same size. Different balls are suitable for differently sized people. The key is being able to sit comfortably on top of the ball with your knees bent and your feet flat on the floor.

Everything you do perched on the ball involves a little bit of balancing, and this means working the muscles that control your core stability, even if all you're doing is sitting on the thing. There are more effective ways to use them, though.

Here's an idea for you

Try a forward roll out. Kneel on the floor in front of your ball and lean forward very slightly to rest your forearms on it with your hands together. Keeping the abs good and tight, gently roll the ball forward until your arms are straight. Hold that for a moment, then roll it back to the start position. Repeat.

Side stretch

Kneel with the ball next to you and your arm resting on it. Now with the leg that's furthest from the ball stretch straight out sideways and gently shift the weight onto the ball so you are draped over it sideways on. The hand that's not on the ball should now stretch up and over your head towards the ball.

Back stretch

Sit on the centre of the ball, feet a little apart. Then very gently walk your feet away so that you lie back and both your back and neck come down to be supported on the ball. You may want to have a hand behind your head to take the weight off your neck until it's resting on the ball. With your feet flat on the floor, now open your arms on each side and feel the stretch across your back.

12. Balls II

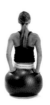

Those over-sized beach balls can also be used for strength work. So forget the fun and games, this is where the balls get their own back.

Swiss balls are inherently unstable, so as you exercise on one you are making minute adjustments all the time in order to keep your balance. With weights in your hands those adjustments are exaggerated, and so your mid section, and in particular the deeply-lying stomach muscles, gets a workout as you work the arms. You can also use yourself as a weight. Here goes:

The push-up
Adopt the standard face-down press-up position, only with your knees on the ball (or your ankles if you're a press-up powerhouse). Now bend your elbows and lower your face towards the floor and straighten to get back up – all slowly and with control. Repeat as often as you would a normal press-up but notice where you can feel the squeeze.

Here's an idea for you

Too easy? Try a wall-hanging reverse crunch. Move the ball to a position near the wall bars so you can lie across the ball with your lower back on it while your hands stretch out above your head to grip the bars. Your legs should be bent with your feet on the floor. Now lift your knees up into your chest as you would with a normal reverse crunch. You'll not only have to lift them but also balance them...

By raising the feet above the level of the floor, you put more of your body weight onto your arms which works the triceps, and the tilt throws the effort more onto the upper part of the chest. Because your feet aren't only raised, but balancing on a ball, you'll also have to correct the wobbles, meaning that you will tense and work your abdominals.

The jack-knife

Assume the press-up position, again with your feet together on the ball, only this time keep your arms straight and bend your knees, gently rolling the ball towards you. Now straighten out your legs to get you and the ball back to where they were. Control is the key here and you should quickly feel that most of the effort is coming from your midsection.

13. Stairway to heaven

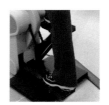

The stepper is how you forge buns of steel, but you can also get a full fat-burning cardio and core-strength workout at the same time. Shhh... here's the secret.

Most people see the stepper as a means of toning the buttocks, and for some reason this means that it is largely left to the women. This is presumably some kind of throwback to the days when men honestly believed that biceps were what attracted the opposite sex.

But the first thing to understand is that stairs are hard work because we are supporting our own body weight and lifting it up, making each step a mini-lunge or squat. Up the resistance of the stepper so you have to launch yourself a little harder and you now have a tough workout for the quads at the front of your thighs and the calves at the back of your legs. Upping the resistance also takes the stepper into serious cardio workout territory. Here's the biggest single

Here's an idea for you

Most people looking to push themselves simply up the resistance, but here's another approach. With the resistance fairly low, try upping the ante by pumping the steps faster, running or pedalling on the spot.

tip of standout stepping. It's breathtakingly simple, little known and changes everything. *Just. Let. Go.*

Give it some and let go, that's all there is to it. You see people hanging off steppers in all sorts of ways, resting their body weight on their arms (bad for the wrists), or hanging off backwards. What you don't see are people who let go and use their arms as counterbalances to their pumping legs.

Let go, and now your legs are taking all your body weight which massively increases the benefits. It forces you to balance, which brings in all the muscles of the torso and builds up core strength. With all your weight on your legs, driving the stepper, you'll burn calories at around twice the rate you get on a stationary bike and not so much less than when you're on the treadmill. Unlike the treadmill, however, the stepper remains a very low-impact activity with minimal shock on the joints.

14. Static crackle

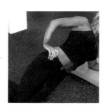

Sit-ups, crunches, reverse crunches – have you ever wondered if there was another way to a strong mid-section without all the bobbing up and down? There is – time to get static.

Movement isn't the only way to build muscle, and that is where isometric exercises come in. Isometrics really mean tensing a muscle without moving anything – either just by contracting it, or by applying a force to something that simply can't go anywhere.

Because it is seen as better to exercise a muscle through its full range of movement, isometric exercises aren't usually recommended for fitness fans unless they've suffered injury to a joint and want to maintain strength. There is, however, an exception – the plank and its variants. The whole point is to hold the body perfectly still, which requires quite a bit of muscular effort because it's only supported on the ground at a couple of points.

Here's an idea for you

Enjoy the side plank but find it too easy? To put a bit of a stretch down the other side of the body, assume the position and stick your 'spare' arm straight out sideways so it points at the ceiling. Now stretch the arm further over your head. Hold the position for as long as you can.

The plank

Lie face down on a mat and then lift up so you are resting your weight on your forearms and your toes (or knees, if toes proves too hard). Now hold that position absolutely rigidly. Your back should be straight – if your bum is sticking up, pull it back into line. If your hips or belly are sagging, then whip them back into line too. You are straight as a ramrod. Keep going for as long as you can – time yourself and see if you can get any better.

The side plank

This time you start on your side and raise yourself onto your elbow with your body dead straight so that there is a long wedge of daylight underneath you from your elbow (which should be directly under your shoulder) right down to your feet. When you can't hold it anymore roll over to your other side and repeat.

15. Back down

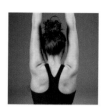

Neglect your back and no one will see your six-pack or admire your navel piercing because you'll be hunched up like Quasimodo doing his shoelaces.

Most muscles have an opposite muscle that's just as important. Most exercises are designed to work both, either in tandem, or one after the other, so as not to create an imbalance. In one key area, however, that rule seems to go out of the window. We tend to forget that unless we strengthen the spinal muscles we could be sowing the seeds of serious back trouble. The more you're working the rest of your body, the more you need a strong back to hold it all together, and the muscles that get ignored are the erector spinae which run up the length of the spine.

Before working your back you should be sure to have sought medical advice and talked it over with the gym instructors. You have? Promise?

Here's an idea for you

Try doing the Superman-style back extension on a Swiss ball. With your feet firmly on the floor, lie face down on the ball so it supports your stomach and ribs. Now lift your head and shoulders off the ball and curve your back upwards.

Superman – or, indeed, Superwoman

Lie flat on your front on a mat and smoothly lift both your arms and your feet off the mat as if you were trying to curl your whole body into a bow shape with only your stomach, ribs and hips left on the mat. Keep it steady, hold for a moment, then return. Now add a slight twist by slowly raising your right arm with your left leg, then your left arm with your right leg. This should be comfortable enough to do ten or twenty times without feeling difficult.

Good morning

Stand with your feet shoulder-width apart and your knees slightly bent. Bend forward from the waist until your torso is parallel to the floor and hold this position for a moment before gently rising back up. If you feel great, you can add weight with either a very light barbell across your shoulders or a light dumbbell in each hand with the weight resting on each shoulder. If you are a beginner to back workouts or feel a twinge, then don't use the weights.

16. On yer bike I: Style

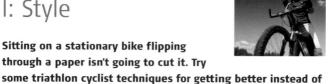

Sitting on a stationary bike flipping through a paper isn't going to cut it. Try some triathlon cyclist techniques for getting better instead of just getting bored.

Time to stop junk training and improve your technique. On the upright bike, make sure you've got the seat adjusted so your knee is very slightly bent at the bottom of the stroke. Sit upright – don't lean forward and rest your weight on your wrists or elbows, and ensure foot-straps are tight.

Most of us think that pedalling is essentially a downwards push, but the pros like to work the pull up as well. This leads to more efficient cycling and recruits more muscles into the stroke, firming up your bum and thighs. There are four parts to the full circle of your pedal cycle:

Here's an idea for you

Once you've got a more efficient stroke, try working one leg at a time. You don't have to take the other foot off the pedal, just be strict about only pushing with one leg. Now try and keep up the revolution count. You'll find that as you get better at working all the way through the stroke you can maintain a higher speed than you did when you used to just push down.

1. *Down* – the bit you're already pushing on.
2. *Bottom and back* – at the bottom of the stroke. You should be pulling back at this point.
3. *Up* – harder without being 'clipped-on' with cycle shoes, but you can still pull on this part if you have those foot-straps done up.
4. *Top* – imagine the curve at this transition point from pulling up to pushing down.

Break the stroke down and try to spend a couple of minutes pushing on stroke 1. Then switch to the second part of the stroke and focus on putting your effort into that. Then the third part, and the fourth. With a bit of practice you should be able to feel a smoother all-round rhythm.

17. On yer bike II: Strength

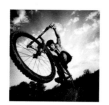

Turn your cycling skills into raw power by looking at strength work.

There are two key parts to this: cadence, which means how fast you're spinning those pedals, and resistance, which is how hard the machine is trying to stop you from spinning those pedals.

Cadence

In cycling terms 'spinning' is a technique in which you choose a gear that means there is little resistance as you turn it, but you keep the speed up so that you're spinning the pedals at high speed (100 r.p.m. and more). For long-distance racing cyclists spinning equates to high speeds over a long period, for time-pressed gym users it can mean harder, but more interesting, workouts.

Resistance

Most stationary bikes these days have a whole smorgasbord of settings and odds are one of them will be called something along the

Here's an idea for you

As you get used to short periods of peak effort with this workout, try to combine it with heart monitoring to see how fast your pulse drops back down from its maximum afterwards. Many stationary bikes have built-in heart monitors or you can use your own.

lines of 'hill climb'. Hill climb programmes on gym bikes vary, but there's usually a choice between a single long steady up and down and a series of short, sharp ups and downs. If you have an option that gives you a series of peaks, then go for that; if not, opt for manual and make your own peaks.

The idea is that the resistance level should leave you feeling comfortable pedalling at the bottom of each 'hill', then working harder as you go up. Right at the top (which should be held for 1–2 minutes) you should feel better if you get up out of the saddle and stand up to pedal. Bingo. As you stand up to pedal try to 'lock' your whole body absolutely steady so you don't bob up and down at all. Try to hold that position for a minute or two, then drop back down (and lower the resistance if necessary). A series of four or five hills each with a standing 'peak' should give you a workout you'll remember.

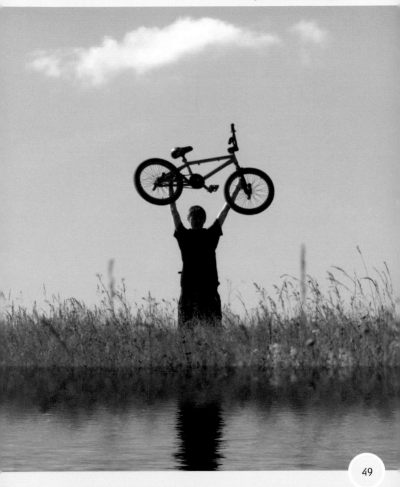

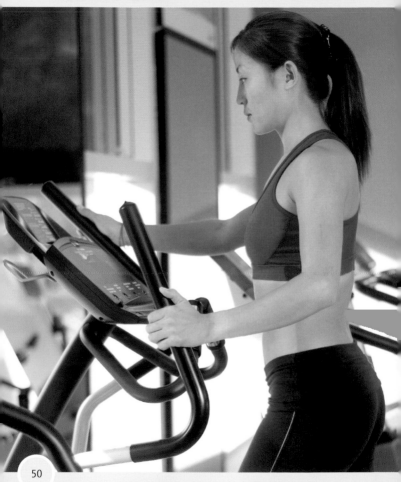

18. Total ellipse

The elliptical trainer is a relatively new kid on the gym block but its popularity means that it's a rare gym without a small posse of them.

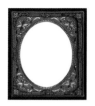

Compared to the other machines in the gym the elliptical trainer has a number of unique advantages. It makes you work with your own bodyweight, but with no impact (your feet never lift off the pedals), and you use your arms. The result is a high calorie burn rate, and an overall workout that makes it a great warm up for other exercises. Ellipticals are low impact and it's hard for you to injure yourself, but try to keep your knees slightly bent at all times; they should never lock. Keep your arms relaxed and try not to bounce your body.

This is a largely self-explanatory machine, with a few variations from one model to another. Pretty much all the machines you'll come across have a resistance setting (usually from 1 to 20) and the higher you set that the more work

Here's an idea for you

Try jogging. Set it to a (very) low resistance level and, watching your balance, let go of the handles. Accelerate slowly and don't outrun the pedals so your feet lift off (which is why you're on very low resistance). Now try to 'run' for two to five minutes before resuming your normal routine.

you'll have to do to keep going. Try different settings to add a bit of variety to your routine.

You have two possible actions with your arms – you can put your energy into pushing away from you, or into pulling towards you. Pushing will exercise your chest (pectoral) muscles and the backs of your arms (triceps), pulling will put more emphasis on your back (lattisimus dorsi or lats) and your biceps. Try mixing and matching with five minutes just pushing, then five minutes just pulling.

Your lower body muscles are working too. Here you can also mix and match by backing up. The smooth elliptical action makes it easy to go into reverse and walk backwards, which then reverses the action on your muscles and works your buttocks more than your thighs. Again try five minutes of each, switching between the two for a more complete body workout.

19. Roman revenge

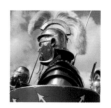

Abs, they say, are made in the kitchen, not in the gym. For most of us the problem with getting a muscular midriff isn't the muscles, it's the fat on top of them.

What if you succeed in burning away that fat only to find that the muscles underneath are more washout than washboard? Most gym goers are already familiar with, and heartily sick of, the crunch, so what else is there to work the abs? Time for the torture apparatus.

Roman chairs come in a variety of shapes but they all look distinctly uncomfortable and have two basic features in common. The first is a padded bar to tuck your lower legs under, and the second is a larger pad to take the weight of your lower body. There are two basic ways of using the chair: face down, which gives you a great back hyperextension (and a view of the floor), and face up, which also gives you a great back hyperextension (and a view of the ceiling).

Here's an idea for you

Not tough enough? Next time, instead of having your hands on your ears as you crunch/hyperextend, try folded across your chest – holding a weight. Take it steady at first but as you build up the load, you'll build up the muscle.

53

Notice that word 'hyperextension'. The point of the Roman chair is that it makes your muscles work through a wider range of movement than usual, and if you have a weak back this could be dangerous. If in doubt, take professional advice.

Make sure you're nicely warmed up and then lie face down, with the backs of your calves tucked under the padded bar, your elbows bent and your hands on your ears. Now smoothly bend your body forwards and extend your shoulders down towards the floor. Equally smoothly bring your body back to horizontal, and then arch upwards so you are lifting your shoulders and chest high off the horizontal. This will work your back muscles but you will also quickly realise that you have to tense your stomach muscles (and your buttocks) to maintain the position. That's a rep. Try ten to twelve more.

20. Hanging around

You've done everything you can to strip the fat off your belly, but what's left underneath isn't quite the toned midsection you see on MTV. What to do?

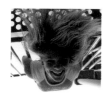

Hanging leg raises can be performed from a chinning bar (the horizontal metal bar set above head height) but you'll probably find it very tiring on the hands. Much better is to look around for a leg-raise 'chair' – sometimes called a Roman chair, but not to be confused with the mutant bench of the same name. The leg-raise chair is a vertical metal frame with a cushioned backrest and support pads to rest your forearms on as they take the weight of your body (your legs hanging freely below).

Having warmed up on something that works upper and lower body (such as an elliptical trainer or a rowing machine), jump up into the chair with your back pressed against the back rest and your weight on your forearms. Step off

Here's an idea for you

Try the bent knees standard leg raise as normal, but as you raise your leg twist your body to the side so that at the end of the movement your feet are sideways on and perpendicular to the floor. Lower gently back to resting position and do the same movement but for the other side. Resist the temptation to swing your legs up.

the foot rests so that your legs are hanging unsupported, then smoothly bend and lift your legs up towards your chest. At the end of the move you should also be tilting your pelvis upwards to get the last part of the lift nice and high. Keeping the whole movement slow and controlled, lower the legs back down to the starting position. That's a rep, try eight to ten more, and see if you can build up from one set of ten to three or four.

To make it harder you can try the exercise with 'straight' legs but don't lock the knees and try to keep them slightly bent. Keep it smooth and controlled at all times, and don't ignore any tightness or strain in your back.

21. At a stretch

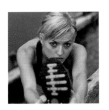

Stretching seems like a pain, so it's probably the first thing to drop off your workout list. Skip the stretching, however, and you increase injury risk and miss out on performance.

Skipping the stretching is one of those naughty little sins we've all been guilty of from time to time. Stretching takes time, it's uncomfortable and it's hard to see the point. Until something goes wrong, of course. But there's more to stretching than just avoiding injury. By gently extending the range of movement in joints and muscles you open up new performance possibilities. Longer strides when running, or strokes when swimming, and better skiing technique are among the potential benefits of extended flexibility.

Stretch steadily, and stretch often, easing into a stretch only to that delicate point where it's edging on discomfort and absolutely not to

Here's an idea for you

Try the three-way stretch. Sit on the floor with one leg straight out in front of you. Bend the other leg, pulling your ankle as far up into your groin as you can with the sole of your foot resting on the upper thigh of the other leg. Now reach down the straight leg as far as you can with both hands. Try not to tense the straight leg. Hold for thirty seconds, gently release and switch legs.

the point where it hurts to hold the stretch. If it hurts, stop at once. You may have heard of ballistic stretching which is highly athletic and active, but leave that to others, just focus on static work for the moment.

Your muscles should be warm when you stretch (don't confuse stretching and warming up) and you should hold the stretch for thirty seconds with up to a minute tops if you're very comfortable. Although the temptation is to head for the shower as soon as you get off the treadmill/stepper/bike it is precisely at that moment, when you're still hot and bothered, that stretching can do the most good.

There's a stretch for every part of your body – including a few you're probably not familiar with yet. Take the time to find out about the stretches specific to your sport, and then take the time to do them.

22. Spring into action

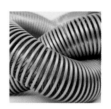

Plyometrics aren't for everyone – their explosive nature means they entail a higher risk of injury than most exercises. They can prepare you, however, for those fleeting seconds of all–or–nothing effort.

The idea behind plyometrics is much like that of a spring. The more you 'load' a spring by pushing down on it, the higher it bounces back when you let go. Similarly you can 'load' a muscle by contracting it 'eccentrically', by lengthening it, then immediately contracting it 'concentrically' (by shortening it). The idea is that you get a boost in the force of the second contraction. It's only to be considered by those already in very good shape. There are a few other sensible precautions:

- Always warm up thoroughly.
- Don't do plyometrics after a strength workout when the muscles are already tired.
- Keep the volume low.
- Give yourself plenty of rest between sessions.

Here's an idea for you

Try step jumps. Set up a step so that it's about a foot high. Step backwards off the top of it so you drop to the ground, then immediately bounce back up to land on the step. If you step backwards, then the jump will be forwards.

■ Cushion the fall. Wear proper sports shoes, avoid concrete floors, use a mat.

Here are some ideas. For your lower body:

Standing jump – Stand with your feet shoulder-width apart. Squat down slightly and immediately explode upwards, reaching both arms up for the ceiling. Take care to land with knees slightly bent to cushion the shock.

Side jump – Start as for the standing jump but this time jump sideways about a foot, landing both feet together. Immediately bounce back again.

For your upper body:

Clap press-up – Take up the normal press-up position, drop down fast, then push up so hard you lift up off the ground, clap your hands together in the air, then get them back into the original position fast enough to catch yourself on the ground. Repeat.

23. The Gravitron

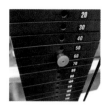

It sounds like something Luke Skywalker would drive, but you'll find that the Gravitron is as clever as it is big when it comes to upper-body workouts.

The idea is simple. Working with your own bodyweight is a great way of building strength and hauling yourself up and down is a natural movement that combines many muscles at once. The Gravitron works by the same sort of weights and pulleys as other weights machines, except that here they are set up as counterbalances acting against your body weight. Which means that the more weight you select on the Gravitron, the less weight you actually have lift to get your body to perform dips and pull-ups. You get the same range of movement as the real thing, but you get to choose just how hard it is to do.

Dips

The triceps and shoulder exercise *par excellence*, dips tone those upper arms a treat. First, set a weight on the Gravitron. Remember that however many kilos it says on the

Here's an idea for you

If you really want to make life tough for yourself, try pull-ups with a towel grip. You may want to counterbalance yourself with more weight than usual as this is much tougher. You'll need two small sweat towels. Drape one over each upper hand rest and take firm hold of the hanging towel ends. Now try to pull up.

metal plate you select, the figure you will lift is your weight minus that figure. The more weight you select, the easier it is for you to complete the exercise. Kneel on the knee pads facing the machine and hold the lower set of hand grips which should be at about waist level. Smoothly lower your body by bending your elbows until your upper arms are parallel with the floor. Straighten your arms to return to your original position. That's a rep.

Pull-ups

The principal muscles worked are the lats of your back, and the biceps as you bend your arms in the last part of the pull. You start exactly as for the dips, but this time reach up for the bars above your head. Pull up until your head reaches at least hand level and let yourself slowly back down. That's a rep.

24. Meeting Mr Smith

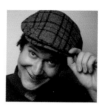

The Smith machine is intimidating, but get to grips with it and you'll find it offers a far more forgiving path into working with weights than the conventional approach.

The Smith machine is basically a barbell trapped in a metal frame so that it can only move straight up and down in a smooth sliding motion. It has hooks on the bar so it can be locked into different resting positions at different heights. To load it, you slide weight plates onto the ends. To work with it, you can set it on a high starting position and stand underneath it for squats or lunges where your legs are doing the work of raising the weight. Alternatively you can position a bench under it and work sitting down, for example doing military presses where you push a weight up from your shoulders to the point where your arms are straight. Another position is to use the bench lying down and bench press your little heart out.

Here's an idea for you

Set up a flat bench and try bench pressing without the need for a spotter's help, or set it up as an incline seat (so the 'back' of the chair slopes backwards) and do incline chest presses. By working at an incline you shift the load onto the shoulders and upper chest.

Because the bar only moves in one direction and one plane you won't develop all the stabilising muscles used for free weights, so serious body builders should stick to barbells. But the Smith machine allows normal mortals to feel much safer using weights because we don't have to worry about becoming unbalanced. Or squashed like a pancake – you don't need a 'spotter' to grab the weight if you get over-ambitious. Simply turning your wrists engages the hook on the next rest point down the rack. If the weight suddenly feels like too much, then a quick twist of the wrist hands it back to the care of Mr Smith.

The Smith machine is not a place to start learning about weights from scratch. If terms like 'bench press', 'squats' or 'lunges' have you furrowing your brow in confusion, then ask an instructor for help or try a pump class.

25. Take it slow

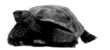

In a hurry to get stronger? *Slow down*. That's the promise of super slow lifting, a technique that promises better results from fewer repetitions and only one or two sessions a week.

Taking it slowly is not to be confused with taking it easy. The approach requires only a few lifts, but each one takes 15–20 seconds consisting of a slow lift, hold and slow descent. Super slow lifting has attracted a following of people who swear that slowing down is vastly superior to speeding up; there is an equal and opposite movement that claims that the benefits are only in the early stages of strength training and don't help the hardcore.

So if you're fairly new to strength training, short of time or looking for something different, then note that the short-term benefits of slow lifting are:

■ It gives a more intensive session within a shorter time.

Here's an idea for you

Try working to muscle failure. Keep going on a weight, just as slowly, until you realise you simply aren't going to manage to lift it all the way for ten seconds. In keeping with the technique, however, remember not to just drop it – even if you can't make the full lift, you should try to slow down the descent just as much as usual.

- It teaches good form; you have to focus on each part of the lift.
- It takes momentum out of the equation so you can't 'cheat' by swinging your way through a set.
- It's less likely to cause injuries through jerky technique.

Which makes it worth a try, especially if you only get to the weights room once a week.

Try this workout.

Squats – Using a barbell, squat machine or Smith machine try a weight you can normally lift comfortably 12–20 times and try for six to eight lifts counting ten seconds up, ten seconds down. That's a rep. Six or seven more of those and that's a wrap.

Bench press – As above, preferably using a Smith machine unless you are confident you can stabilise a barbell for such a long lift (and have a spotter to watch over you).

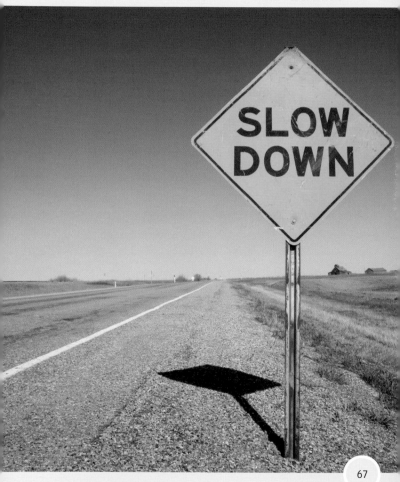

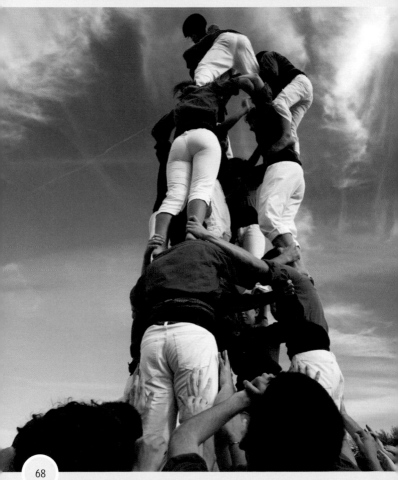

26. Pyramid power

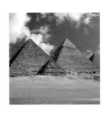

Lifting weights and pushing iron quickly gets boring – both for you and your muscles. To keep both you and your body on its toes, try varying the routine a little.

There's nothing that complicated about pyramid sets. You start with lighter weights and more repetitions, then increase the weights and decrease the repetitions with each set. Starting with 'light and lots' helps stretch and warm the muscles before you hit them with the heavy stuff and so helps prevent injury. Us men in particular tend to enjoy pyramid sets because we're forever trying to play with heavier dumbbells or notch the machine up one more number than before. The pyramid system means that the final set is probably using a heavier weight than we could manage in the classic approach (albeit for fewer repetitions), so we get to walk away from the machine feeling well chuffed.

Here's an idea for you

For the full pyramid you don't stop with the third set of heavier weights but instead continue back down the pyramid, doing further sets with lighter weights and higher repetitions. Rather than ending up doing five or more sets, try doing the normal pyramid set, ending on your heaviest weights and lifting those to failure (i.e. you can't complete that last lift). Then drop the weight down by a couple of notches and lift ten more of the lighter weight.

69

Try this pyramid set with dumbbells – please note that these weights are just for guidance, if you're built like a carthorse then you'd need to up the weight. Try doing curls, standing in front of the mirror, and using a 'hammer' grip so that when your arm is at the top of the lift the weight is vertical in your hand, as if you were holding a hammer. Don't move your upper body or shoulder to help with the exercise.

- Set 1 – 1 kg dumbbell, 12 reps
- Set 2 – 1.5 kg dumbbell, 10 reps
- Set 3 – 2 kg dumbbell, 8 reps

The same principle can be applied to any of the weight machines, the Smith machine or the free weights.

27. Try a tri

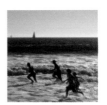

Triathlons are popular but seem to need a lot of organisation, kit and time. Doing your own in the gym, however, is easy, convenient and doesn't even have to involve getting wet.

Unlike traditional long-distance events, triathlon breaks up the race into three disciplines that work different parts of the body in different ways. The wonders of the gym, however, mean you can not only try a tri, but compete against your friends, and all without buying equipment, or even having to swim.

The full Olympic triathlon distance is a 1.5 km swim, a 40 km cycle and a 10 km run but most people start with either a 'sprint' distance of 750 m swim, 20 km cycle and 5 km run, or even a 'super sprint' which is half that distance again. Start small and work upwards. Outside, the swim always comes first, but for your indoor triathlon you may want to make the swim last as a way of cooling down. It's

Here's an idea for you

You can substitute the rowing machine for the swim. There is even a well-known triathlon that starts on a rowing machine before charging outdoors for the ride and run. The distance is 4000 m on a Concept II rowing machine, a 25 km cycle and 7.5 km run.

still a good idea to do the cycle before the run as it's an efficient and non-impact way of warming up.

Having decided your distance, you now have to complete it. First off will be the stationary bike for the distance you have set. Make a note of the time taken but also the resistance level as it will be useful for comparing your performance in the future.

Then comes the treadmill. You're already warmed up, so you can get stuck in at your normal running speed for the distance you've set yourself. Again note your time and the incline you used, then off to the changing rooms and into the pool.

Triathlon swimmers race freestyle (i.e. front crawl) but the rules allow any kind of stroke so don't feel obliged to crawl unless that's what you're comfortable with.

28. Mystery muscles

Here are a few moves especially for the sinews that slipped your mind. You can point to your abs... but what about your obliques, transversus and erector spinae?

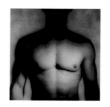

We all want toned tummies, and we've all crunched away to get them – but the crunch only really works the rectus abdominis muscle. You've also got to pay attention to the external and internal obliques and the transversus abdominis.

■ *Obliques – Swiss ball Russian twist*
The obliques work together down the sides of the abdomen and take care of turning motions. Crunches with a twist (right arm to left knee for example) will work them; try sitting on a Swiss ball for variety.

Walk your legs away forwards so that you are left with your hips and lower torso on the ball. Now lift your shoulders up and forwards and with your arms extended straight out twist your upper body sideways to the left, the centre, again, then the right. Repeat.

Here's an idea for you

Working on stronger arms often focuses on upper arms at the expense of forearm strength. Try wrapping a sweat towel around the bar or hand grips when lifting to make the grip bigger and work the wrist and forearm muscles more.

■ *Transversus – abdominal breathing*

A strong and taut transversus not only armour-plates your midriff but flattens it. Lie flat on your back and place the flat of your hand on your stomach. Now breathe in deeply for a count of four, breathing from your stomach – imagine drawing that diaphragm deep down towards your pelvis. Expel the air for eight counts by compressing your stomach muscles, then hold that muscle pressed against your spine for a minute and try to breathe normally without letting it relax.

■ *Erector spinae – cable row*

These are the muscles that pull your spine straight. Overdoing it on the abs can tighten up your stomach and weaken the pull of the erector spinae, leading to back trouble. Rowing machines will help, but you could try a cable row. This will feature a seat, a foot plate and a low pulley with a cable and handle. Sit on the seat and holding the handle in both hands row it back towards you just as you would a rowing machine (but without the legs).

29. Step up a gear

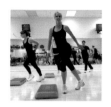

The choreography of step may look daunting but give it a try. It's a full-on cardio workout to music that firms the thighs, shapes the bum and hones the hamstrings.

When step was first introduced it was billed as 'the workout with muscle'. Unlike all that aerobics skipping around that went before it, step introduced high repetition strength moves. This also made it slightly more acceptable to men.

Steps of any kind are a surprisingly hard workout – just ask anyone who doesn't live and work in a bungalow. Stepping up and down for an hour is a thorough cardio workout and is only made possible by a careful mix of different moves and motivating music. Spend a few minutes watching a step class of regulars, everyone beat perfect, stomping their way through their favourite numbers and you'll witness a semi-mystical rite more normally associated with shamans and dervishes.

Here's an idea for you

Most gyms have several levels of step to help keep you on your toes, and you should progress to the next one (intermediate or advanced) as appropriate. In practice, that means as soon as you find that you know what comes next, you're not as breathless or sweaty as you used to be, or you just fancy something new.

Make sure you start with a beginners' class: step is hard enough work without the stress of playing catch-up. You'll probably warm up with some nice simple side-to-side movements, a bit of stretching as you sway, and some step up/downs. Then the pace will gradually pick up with new moves being added such as stepping sideways on the step, stepping down on the other side, stepping over the step with a twirl to face the other way. The whole thing is done to a strong beat – you'll find the effect a little like slow-motion morris dancing with added leotards. You may be surprised by how much you sweat. Step is one of those things where it gets easier the better you get at it. As a newbie you are putting in more effort, and getting more of a workout, than the more slick-looking steppers around you.

30. Hard core

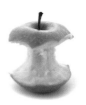

Why would you get in line to play with a wobble board with springs? Because you can tone your tum, boost your balance and build your fitness, that's why.

The core board is a development of the old wobble board – a board with half a football stuck on the bottom. By adding springs, the core board gives you the instability of the wobble board, but also fights back by trying to return itself to where it wants to be just as you are trying to get it to go somewhere else. The result is that you get to build up the stabilising and balancing muscles of your torso. And fall off from time to time, naturally.

If you try to rotate your body in a vertical axis the core board will try to push you back the other way. To combat that you have to use muscular force to counter the turning action as well as keep your balance. It makes for a varied and active workout but is still quite gentle – it was created to help rehabilitate injured football players. Not only does the board help build up core strength by recruiting as

Here's an idea for you

Getting particularly confident on the basic balances? OK, just for a moment try shutting your eyes as you do them. It should throw you off enough to make it interesting without sending you careering across the studio.

many muscles as possible to help balance, it also gently 'surprises' your muscles with its twists, strengthening them and making them much less likely to be shocked or injured when you make a desperate lunge.

You start off with some stretches to loosen the hamstrings, hip flexors and calves, then a few simple balances on the board. Next you move on to a little bit of rhythmic movement interrupted with stationary balances. Expect to spend a fair amount of time on the end of the board with one leg in the air doing squats and delivering slow motion (and very wobbly) kicks sideways, forwards and backwards. Then you'll move on to a bit of upper body and obliques work, possibly kneeling on the floor with one arm balanced on the board and twisting away for all you're worth.

31. Mortal combat

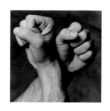

Mixing martial arts moves and music is a trend sweeping gyms worldwide. Work off some aggression along with the pounds.

It's a rare gym these days that doesn't feature body combat, tae box or another exotically named equivalent. For a lot of people aggressive workouts work.

BodyCombat is the trademark name of the workout from the Les Mills company (the guys who brought you BodyPump) and if your gym isn't a subscriber then it's likely to have another flavour with a different name but much the same moves. These are taken from boxing, tai chi, kickboxing and tae kwondo, choreographed into pumping, all-dancing, all-kicking extravaganzas. Even though they are billed as non-contact that doesn't mean they are no-impact for your body. The bouncing up and down, sudden changes of direction and shooting your limbs out in various directions are all exhilarating but hard on the joints. You'll need to be in fairly good shape, and wearing shoes with good ankle support.

Here's an idea for you

Martial arts moves are hard on the body because they require both simple endurance and explosive movements. To get better you will need to work on cardio endurance – try the treadmill.

Ask at your gym if any of the courses with martial arts moves actually involve contact pads, then trot along and try it. With contact versions of martial arts workouts you still warm up by heaving punches and launching kicks at the atmosphere, but you then move on to trying to land them on someone. This isn't as painful as it sounds. You'll be divided up into pairs and one of you holds the pad while the other launches attacks on it. Padded gloves protect the puncher's pandies. Hand pads can be held horizontally for you to deliver upper cuts to, or vertically to practice jabs. Full body pads can be held up to act as targets for kicks or hooks. You'll get to take turns at holding or hitting the pads, and holding them can be more of a workout than you expect.

32. Food and drink

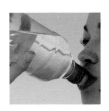

Eating and drinking may have led you to the gym but now's not the time to stop. The trick is to know what to eat and drink before, during and after training.

These recommendations are aimed at those doing cardio/calorie-burning exercises. The standard wisdom in the body-building world is that you can burn fat, or you can build muscle, but trying to do both at once is counterproductive. You're better off burning fat first before moving on to muscling up.

Before

If you head for the gym before work, the usual recommendation is a light breakfast based on carbohydrates (like cereals). Breakfast bars and sports bars can provide a good balance but be careful because a lot of breakfast bars have a very high fat content and sports bars are high calorie. Many people find it hard to stomach anything before a workout. It's probably more important to consider what you shouldn't eat, rather than what

Here's an idea for you

Make sure you take a large drinking bottle with you to the gym and keep it to hand whenever you're in a class or on a machine. If bag space is a problem, then go to a camping shop and get a fold-flat polythene drinking pouch that you can roll up when it's empty.

you should. Big no-nos include sugar – you'll get a high followed later by a low – and protein, which is hard to digest.

During
Drink! In the course of an hour's intense exercise you can lose two pounds of bodyweight. Those two pounds are all water and if you don't put this back into your system your cells malfunction and your blood volume decreases. So drink, but to rehydrate in a hurry you should opt for so-called isotonic sports drinks.

After
Eat. You want to avoid the energy trough that can follow a workout because your long-term motivation is going to be a lot better if you end up feeling great. Also the body is complex, and if you make huge energy demands on it and then don't feed it you may be sending the wrong messages. It may even try to hold on to fat reserves.

33. Pump that body

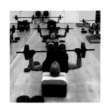

Hanker after muscle tone? Prefer your exercise to be set to music with clear instructions? That doesn't sound so unreasonable, in fact it sounds a lot like BodyPump.

BodyPump came from New Zealand in 1990 and has proved an instant hit worldwide because it answers an obvious need. Lots of us are looking for more toned upper bodies, we've come to realise that cardio work and normal aerobics aren't going to do the job, and the macho atmosphere of the weights room can be a serious turn off.

By combining barbells and bench (in the form of an aerobics step) the BodyPump routine is designed to give a complete body workout. On the way it gives you an idea of all the most common weights moves – squats, lunges, bench press, shoulder press, curls, etc. First there's a warm-up, then the big muscle groups and combinations are worked with squats, bench press and back work. Then it moves on to focus on

Here's an idea for you

The squat is often a problem area in pump for those worried about their back. Try this front squat: place the bar across the front of your shoulders in front of your neck. Cross your arms to give more stability on the grip. Front loading can help keep your spine neutral.

smaller muscles like biceps and triceps, the shoulders and finally the abs and a cool-down and stretch. It's pretty much a lesson in good workout procedure. By using light weights (which the user chooses) and high repetitions the aim is very much on toning, not on building muscle.

Look around in a pump class and you'll see that a lot of those working away are women – which is the hallmark of BodyPump's success. It's clear what to do, the basic pattern stays the same, the instructor is there to show you and the whole thing is set to thumping music to keep the blood up. Nor is it just 'weights lite' for newbies – it's a pretty good all-round workout for anyone interested in toning. Because it uses free weights and thus recruits the balancing muscles, and because it imposes the discipline of working all the main muscle groups, it's a lot more thorough than most of those hesitant sessions you see people putting in on the fixed weight machines.

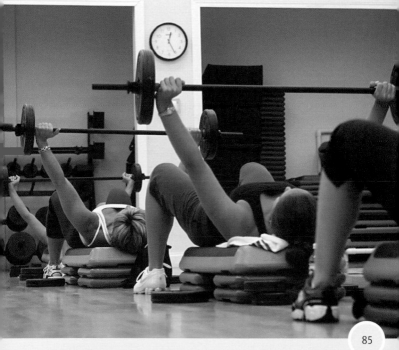

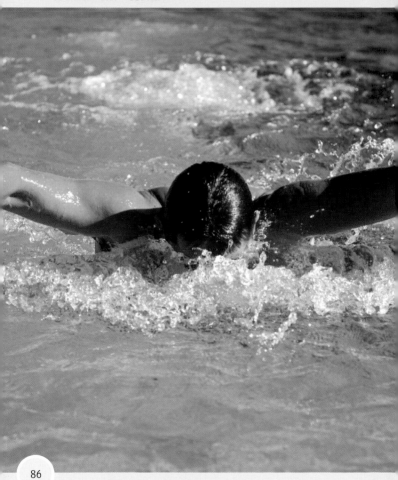

34. In the swim I

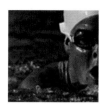

Swimming is one of the best all-round exercises known but most of us, if we're honest, are no better at swimming than we were at school. Learn to cut a dash as you splash.

Swimming involves your whole body. It works your heart and lungs, it increases strength, flexibility and endurance, but involves very little risk of injury. It is often picked out as one of the few exercises where even a very hard workout leaves you feeling good and ready for the rest of the day.

It can be hard to make progress; the default option is just to flounder up and down a bit. Swimming involves a fairly complex set of movements and rhythms and it sometimes helps to break them down in order to focus on individual elements. Here we're going to focus on just the arm, and then just the leg movements in isolation. You'll remember the

Here's an idea for you

Swim a length and count the number of strokes it takes. Using what you've learned from swimming with arms or legs only, try to swim the length using fewer strokes. See how far you can bring down your score by concentrating on getting the most progress out of the fewest number of strokes.

humble float from your days as a learner. The pull-buoy may be less familiar but basically it's just a float that's shaped so it's easier to hold between your legs.

Legs

Scissors kick, butterfly kick or frog-leg strokes should all be enough on their own to propel you from one end of the pool to the other. Grab a float, hold it out in front of you with both hands and use only your legs to swim.

Arms

As with legs, only in reverse. Lodge a pull buoy or a float (you may need two depending on your natural buoyancy or lack of it) between your thighs. Now set off up the pool using only your arm stroke.

In both of these cases the aim is not to be fast, but to be comfortable. If you are tired after a length, then you may want to work on putting less effort into the stroke, and instead improve your form.

35. In the swim II

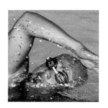

Style is everything in swimming. Good style means ease, speed and the confidence to keep on going for hour after hour.

Trying to go faster by throwing more effort at it will get you nowhere; it's all down to drag. The faster you move through water, the greater the drag created by your body displacing the water as you go. The answer is to streamline your body and reduce the drag.

Think about your posture in the water and try to swim more like a fish and less like a labrador. That means no more looking forwards (which presents your face to the water) but instead looking down and trying to make your whole body like a spear, with your head and spine in line.

The other area where our posture often works against us is that we allow our hips to sink into the water. Thanks to our lungs, our chest cavities are a buoyant floatation aid stuck between our

Here's an idea for you

Total immersion is the coaching philosophy of Terry Laughlin who has set up an entire business around the principle that the key to good swimming is to make yourself more streamlined. Total immersion classes tend to be a bit pricey but the approach had had a lot of success with adult swimmers. Check it out.

shoulders. In order to position our whole bodies higher in the water (so reducing drag) the best approach is to try and push the chest, rather than the hips, into the water so that the buoyancy forces us up.

Although most of us see swimming as something you do on your front or your back, we are actually most streamlined when tilted onto our sides and that's how we should swim front crawl. Instead of keeping your body flat in the water and turning your head right round to breathe at every stroke, try rolling your entire torso with the stroke. You should turn sideways with your pulling arm going deep and your head barely needing to turn at all to clear the water and suck in the air. It's a great technique for those who get neck ache from turning their heads high to get their mouths out of the water.

36. Perfect Pilates

The ballerinas' secret for long and lean muscles is now recognised as having benefits for everyone from recovering rugby players to recovering couch potatoes.

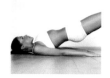

Joseph H. Pilates was no ballerina. A puny youth who suffered from rickets, asthma and rheumatic fever, he developed his famous technique in an attempt to overcome his own weaknesses. His theories have been taken up and moved on by generations of practitioners, but certain characteristics and the basic principles remain unchanged. The keys are concentration, precise control of movement, an understanding of the role and technique of breathing, and of the importance of building a strong physical core to anchor all other movements and exercise.

You start with mat work and perhaps a large sausage of plastic foam. Initially a lot of work will focus on making you aware of specific parts of your body and in particular the muscles of your stomach and the bones you sit on.

Here's an idea for you

Plenty of Pilates practitioners have seized on the Swiss ball as an exercise tool. Doing Pilates on a ball gives you the opportunity to stretch further than before while still being comfortably supported. It's also oddly soothing. Give it a go.

Next come simple movements such as rolling up into a sitting position or lifting legs and shoulder blades off the deck. The moves are all done slowly, with emphasis on breathing correctly, and repetitions are very few. If that sounds a bit cushy, then think again. The degree of concentration, plus the effort of tensing muscles in unfamiliar ways, makes for surprisingly hard work. It also promotes a general feeling of well-being due to measured breathing, gentle pace and the sense of muscle control. That control is also the key to why it appeals so much to recovering athletes.

Among the benefits of Pilates are a greater attention to the deeper-lying muscles of the core, such as the transversus which lies under the abs. For athletes, this core strength approach gives greater balance and power, and there are those who swear that it improves posture so much that you can end up taller!

37. Interval training

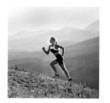

You've probably heard of exercises being either aerobic or anaerobic... but they can be both. Blend them, and you can burn calories and push yourself through an exercise plateau.

Exercise that encourages heart and lungs to work harder and get stronger is known in gym-speak as cardio(vascular), but all such exercise can also be described as aerobic. Aerobic exercise is all about getting air into the body and getting the oxygen from it pumped around as efficiently as possible. Anaerobic exercise is the stuff that happens so fast, so intensely, that the body can't supply the oxygen needed and your muscles have to do without. Anaerobic exercise is all about short sharp shocks. Intense bursts of sprinting are anaerobic, gentle jogging is aerobic.

Mix aerobic and anaerobic and your normal workout becomes more challenging and you get a more intense workout out of a shorter period of time. It also

Here's an idea for you

If you're using a machine that has settings for different workouts, then look for one that regularly raises and decreases the resistance (probably called a 'hill climb'). Instead of slowing down as the machine raises the resistance, set yourself a goal of a certain speed,. Then treat the lower resistance intervals as rests.

makes a change from a routine, and there's evidence that anaerobic exercise increases HGH (human growth hormone) levels, and HGH has anti-ageing properties. So what do you do?

Pick a cardio machine, any machine. Now start off with a nice easy pace and if you or your chosen machine happen to be sporting a heart monitor, try and keep your heart rate at a nice gentle 55–70% of your maximum. After a good 10 minutes of warm-up you're ready to up the level to 70–85% of your maximum heart rate, the optimum for developing cardio efficiency. Five minutes of that and you can go for it with an anaerobic sprint. This means taking it up to a level of effort so intense that 20 seconds is enough to wipe you out. At which point you drop back to your easy level for 5 minutes of active recovery.

38. Timesaving tips

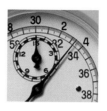

Too pressed for time to have time for presses? Try a few of these tips to maximise those fleeting moments in the gym.

How can you make sure you get a decent workout when you only have a few precious minutes to dedicate to the temple of toning? Try the following.

Have your kit ready, packed up, and by the door. When you pull stuff out of the dryer match it up into complete sets of kit, then make sure you have a gym bag ready to go for every day. Leave it sitting by the door and it will be both convenient to grab and a helpful reminder to your conscience.

Plan your workout. Be clear in advance what your workout goals are. Don't fix on a single machine – it may be in use – but decide in advance how much cardio you're

Here's an idea for you

We spend half our time in the weights room waiting for someone else to get off the machine we want. Meanwhile there's a rack of dumbbells sitting unused in front of a mirror somewhere. Learn the range of dumbbell exercises and you'll be able to get a whole upper-body workout without moving from the spot.

going to do or what weight session you have in mind. Try going early. Working out before the day gets its claws into you means you start out feeling good and get your metabolism up and running. There are also fewer people.

Don't rest, cross-train. Your gym tells you to spend no more than 20 minutes on a machine? Fine, just leap straight off it and onto another. Take ten on each if you like. Forty minutes working on a mix of rower/treadmill/bike will give you a more thorough workout. It uses different muscles and psychologically allows you to put more effort because you know you're changing soon.

The normal practice if you're doing weights is to rest at least 30 seconds in between sets. Don't. Instead switch straight to an exercise that works the opposite set of muscles and cut to and fro between the two with no rest time at all. For example, if you're working biceps, then alternate with a triceps press.

39. Smart dumbbells I

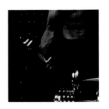

There's more to dumbbells than biceps curls. Combined with some simple accessories, like a bench and your body, they offer one of the most effective workouts. Plus, no queue.

Dumbbells offer more range of movement than any other weights apparatus (you try waving a barbell over your head with one hand) and are also great for chest, abs, legs and back. Here are some moves for your arms, shoulders and chest.

Arms
It would be churlish not to mention the biceps curl so – just as a reminder – stand feet shoulder width apart, don't move your shoulder, and keep the smooth control on both lift and descent. For a bit of variety try a hammer grip in which you hold the dumbbell so it's vertical in your hand at the top of the lift, as if hefting a hammer.

Here's an idea for you

Enjoying the weights work and want to get a bit fancy? Most of these moves can be done swapping the bench for the Swiss ball to add a little imbalance to the move and bring the core muscles of the midsection into the action. Don't be tempted to start off with overly heavy dumbbells.

Triceps time. Standing up, hold the dumbbell in one hand, straighten your arm above you and then gently bend your elbow so the weight comes to rest just behind your neck. Now, without moving anything but your forearm at the elbow, straighten and relax the arm to work the triceps.

Shoulders
With a light weight in each hand, stand with feet shoulder width apart and knees slightly bent and arms by sides. Now lift both arms out straight to the side up to shoulder height. Relax and lift again but this time with arms straight up to the front so you end up in the classic 'sleepwalker' position. Repeat. Lots.

Chest
Try the close-grip bench press. Take a dumbbell in each hand and lie on a bench. Extend both arms straight up above your chest. Lower the weights with your elbows sliding past your sides and stop before the dumbbells reach your chest itself. Repeat.

40. Smart dumbbells II

Dumbbells aren't just for arms. Here's how hand-held weights can work your thighs, hamstrings, calves and buttocks.

You don't need huge weights to work the larger muscles, just good technique and some dumbbells.

Squats

Start with two dumbbells (you can go fairly heavy on this one), one in each hand, at your sides, your feet shoulder width apart, knees very slightly bent. Keep the whole movement smooth and controlled. No bouncing. No grunting. With your shoulders pulled back, bend your knees and ease your body down as if you were slipping into a comfy chair. Don't go so far down that either your knees move further forward than your toes, or your bum is so low that your thighs dip down instead of being parallel to the floor. Go too low and you risk over-extending and straining your muscles. Smoothly raise yourself back up to the start position.

Here's an idea for you

If you lose your balance lunging, check your feet aren't in line. Make sure there is a good 15 cm (6 inches) horizontal difference between the two. To get that, start your lunge with your feet side by side, then step firmly sideways with the foot that is going to go back before stepping backwards into position.

The lunge

Start as with the squat, but this time take a long step forward so your front foot is now about a yard from your back one. Keeping your torso bolt upright, lower your body by bending your legs. Your front knee shouldn't go past your toes (this is a sensible precaution for most exercises or stretches where you bend your knees). Even though you may feel a burning sensation down the length of your back leg it's the muscles of the front thigh that should be doing the work as you now lift your body back up by straightening the front leg.

For a bit of variety, and to hit the calf muscles more, switch from forward lunges – where you step forwards with one leg before lunging – to ones where you step backwards instead.

41. Personal trainers

Personal trainers – fashion accessory for the cash-rich and time poor? Or failsafe route to fitness?

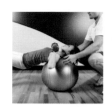

Most gyms these days offer personal training as part of their portfolio. Let's be clear about what a personal trainer means. We're not talking about having someone knock up a tailored training routine for you when you first start – all gyms should do that. Personal trainers will dedicate themselves to you and you alone for each hour that you book. They should assess your fitness level, set up a program complete with goals and waypoints, and provide the motivation to achieve them.

If you're thinking of opting for personal training, ensure that the trainer has a recognised personal trainer qualification, is a member of the Register of Fitness Professionals and has a valid CPR (cardio-pulmonary resuscitation) certificate. Recognised qualifications (as defined by the Register of Fitness Professionals)

Here's an idea for you

If you can't afford a personal trainer, or are a good self-starter who's just short on ideas or direction, then try an online personal trainer. They can supply ideas and help you monitor your own progress. Try GymUser (www.gymuser.co.uk), HandBag (www.handbag.com), or the likes of www.onlinepersonaltrainer.co.uk.

include: Future Fit Training Personal Trainer, YMCA Personal Trainer Diploma, Lifetime HF Personal Trainer, FIE Certified Personal Trainer, Premier Training Diploma or a BA-level degree in sports and fitness.

If you have a clear idea of your fitness targets, the knowledge of how to hit them and a high level of self-motivation, then you don't need a trainer. If, however, you find that motivation is a big problem, or you have an unusual target (say a new sport), or you're going nowhere and don't know what to try, then a personal trainer could be exactly what the doctor ordered.

If your aim is to lose weight and tone up, then you can expect to start off with a cardio warm-up before going onto weights and moves that you wouldn't normally do. In the process you will learn a lot, and a personal trainer can also be a kind of external conscience nagging you if you let things slip.

42. Water workouts

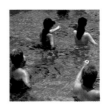

Exercising in water takes twelve times more energy than moving in air. Water also supports your body and makes impact injuries all but impossible.

The wonder of aquatic exercise is that the buoyancy reduces the weight-bearing stress on your joints. It's ideal for everyone from arthritis sufferers to marathon runners suffering from overuse injuries. Heart rates are lower than equivalent land-based activities, but strength gains tend to be higher due to the constant fight against water resistance. Water work is a great workout for endurance, strength and flexibility – so don't dismiss it.

You can expect a friendly, relaxed atmosphere in classes. Basic moves of walking, jumping sometimes with the addition of water 'weights' or 'dumbbells'. The

Here's an idea for you

If you fancy trying water running you don't have to have a deep end and a flotation device to hand. If you can get a moment when the pool isn't packed, try walking or running up and down the lanes of the pool to get a feel for the resistance. If you can 'run' in water up to your thighs, then so much the better – try to concentrate on lifting your knees high with every step.

difference between water weights and land weights is that the water versions are made of foam so that they're buoyant – the effort comes from stopping them rising rather than lifting them up.

The only 'serious' male athletes who have cottoned on to this are runners, for whom water running is now an established technique. Water running requires a flotation device to keep you upright in the water. Other than that you try to 'run' normally but it's exhausting and works your upper body much more than traditional running.

One word of advice whether you are water running or taking part in an aqua aerobics session. Just because you are in water don't think you won't dehydrate. These exercises are deceptive: you don't think you're doing calorie-burning exercise because it feels so gentle, and you have no idea that you are working up a sweat because you're in a pool. Make sure you take a water bottle to your pool workout.

43. Wild workouts

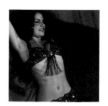

The good workout is the one you keep coming back for... and that means keeping it fun. Gyms are increasingly offering classes that emphasise the play value alongside the carb-burning.

Belly dancing

As an exercise belly dancing is a relatively gentle, low-impact aerobic session with a great deal of emphasis on hip movements which help tone midsections and, in particular, the obliques. It can be much more of a workout than you might think, as it works the stomach, hips and back.

Pole dancing

Pole dancing is erotic dancing using a small stage and a vertical pole that runs from floor to ceiling. As a workout it's the answer to those who love dance-based exercise but worry about upper-body strength. Because the pole moves largely involve

Here's an idea for you

If your gym doesn't go in for anything more exotic than an abs class, then maybe think about joining classes outside the gym or trying a session/day membership at another gym. Some gyms, such as GymBox, specialise in the more fun or off-beat activities, while other specialists such as Circus Space (www.thecircusspace.co.uk) focus on performing arts skills.

grabbing the pole and swinging around it, there's a lot of emphasis on arm and oblique strength. More advanced moves, like swinging upside down and holding the pose, work wonders for core strength and abs. I'm told the atmosphere is a riot. Watch out for friction burns in unlikely places.

Trapeze

Trapeze involves a tough upper-body workout but also a great deal of flexibility and stabilising work. The experts at Circus Space in London also swear that it leads to great posture. Mainly, though, it's a buzz.

Kangoo jumping

Kangoo boots feature a spring (leaf, rather than coil, for any exercise engineers) on the sole which gives a bounce to the step. The class is a warm-up followed by aerobic moves with added boing. Currently the preserve of the more self-consciously groovy gyms.

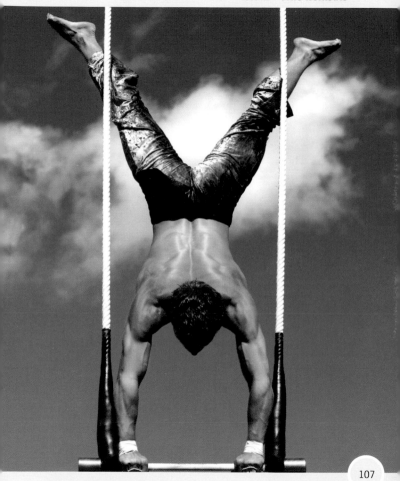

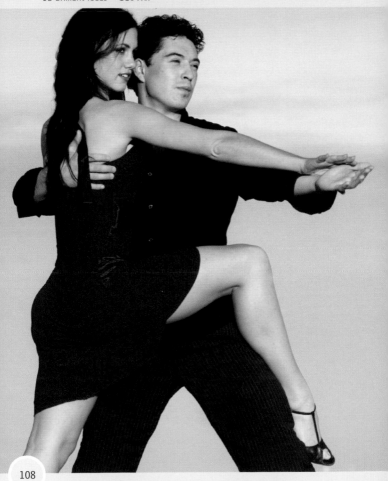

44. Shimmy yourself svelte

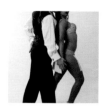

If your gym has just one dance class, then odds on it will be salsa. Here's why.

Salsa is smooth, sexy, but because it's based on relatively simple moves it can be learnt quite quickly (and then improved on forever). As an aerobic workout salsa is low impact – and gets lower as you get better because the weight is kept on the ball of the foot in an elastic movement that cushions the step. It also works up more of a sweat than you might expect; men tend to have a harder time of it, which has the bonus that they get a more thorough workout.

Classes don't normally start with an exercise workout as such but with a refresher of the most basic steps. They then rapidly move on to partner work. Don't worry if you didn't bring a partner; in a typical class everybody will be rotated, dancing with everyone else.

Here's an idea for you

A lot of salsa clubs offer a deal combining a lesson and a night on the tiles. You show up for an hour or so before the club opens and have a refresher lesson, or perhaps learn a new move. By the time the club fills up you'll be much less self-conscious and ready to show off.

Here are a few pointers:

■ In salsa you avoid having the weight on your heels – you always step on the ball of your foot whether going forwards or backwards. It keeps you lighter on your feet, and more mobile.

■ When things speed up, through confidence or a shift in the tempo, remember to make life easier by making your steps smaller.

■ Even though the hip movement is often the slickest aspect of the dance it is not a separate skill from the leg moves. Focus on the steps and the hips will follow when you are relaxed enough to let the rhythm take over.

■ Relax your body and keep your eyes firmly fixed on your partner's face. Start to think too much about your feet and they themselves will forget what comes next.

45. In a spin

If stationary bikes leave you cold but you still like the idea of long lean legs and buttocks like balled-up fists, then it's time to brave the Spinning studio.

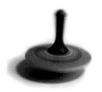

Spinning is a trademark, by the way, so you may find it under a number of other aliases, but you can tell if you're in the right place the moment you swing a leg over the saddle. Start to turn the pedals and you'll realise that they are connected directly to a heavy flywheel. You spin, it spins. The trick is to remember that, unlike a bicycle, if you stop, it doesn't. To slow it down you have to press a knob that pushes a brake pad against the flywheel. To make life harder you have a control to increase the drag against the flywheel so it takes more effort to keep the pedals spinning around.

Spinning classes start with some nice easy warm-up exercises to get you used to the feel of the bike, and to give you an idea of what's in store. There are three basic

Here's an idea for you

Of all the classes you've ever done this is the one where you must have a water bottle to hand. The latest spin bikes have a water holder on the handlebars or frame, the older ones aren't that far from the floor so just stop every now and again (remember to brake the flywheel before it yanks your foot off) and glug.

moves – sprints, climbs and jumps. Sprints are exactly what they sound like; climbs mean a high level of resistance and standing on the pedals to keep it moving. Jumps mean short, sharp spells out of the saddle.

There'll be stomping music – the emphasis is on an all-singing, all-dancing total absorption into the moment and the result is good, sweaty, cardio fun. If you're worried that the pace is likely to be too hectic for you, don't be. It's up to you how much you increase the resistance – your instructor's legs may spin like a washing machine but that doesn't mean you should follow suit straight away.

46. Skipping

Small girls know that skipping is fun. Big, brutish boxers know that skipping is really tough. Somewhere in between there's something for everyone.

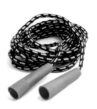

Skipping is a great way to increase stamina, improve co-ordination and tone muscles. It's a huge calorie burner – for a 75 kg man think about 750 calories per hour. It gives much of the workout of running with far less impact. It can be as complex or as simple as you like and, while it takes a few sessions to perfect, it can be done by anybody.

If your gym doesn't have skipping ropes, it has a place to skip and you can bring your own rope. When buying one, look for those with a plastic rope and soft foam handles. Make sure that the handles will stay still in your hands while the rope turns. Select one that's the right size – when you're standing in the middle of it, each

Here's an idea for you

Try a boxer's workout. Skip for three minutes (the time of a round) then perform as many crunches as you can for a minute. Now skip for three minutes again, then perform as many press-ups as you can in a minute. Skip again for three minutes, then a minute of crunches. Repeat until you've worked out for half an hour.

end should reach up to your armpits. If it's too long, knot it; too short, get another.

Make sure you're wearing shoes meant for bounding up and down – that means cross-trainers or basketball shoes but not running shoes – and stretch before you skip. Try to avoid skipping on concrete or a floor laid directly on concrete.

The basic skip step is the pogo with both feet bouncing off the ground together as the rope passes under. Try to keep the weight light on the balls of your feet and make sure you've got good rhythm before trying to increase the speed.

When you begin, aim for short bursts of 20 seconds or so before taking a brief break (a good time to stretch) and then repeating. Build up slowly until you can leave out the breaks and skip for five minutes or more straight. Once you're there it's time to get fancy with the footwork.

47. Hi Lo and BodyAttack

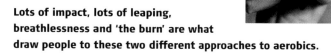

Lots of impact, lots of leaping, breathlessness and 'the burn' are what draw people to these two different approaches to aerobics.

BodyAttack and Hi Lo both work on the same principle (loud music, lots of calorie expenditure) and the benefits are improved circulation, stronger heart and lungs, lower cholesterol and increased bone density (providing you don't break any in the process).

BodyAttack follows the tried and trusted format of other Les Mills exercise routines (such as BodyPump) which means that you warm up and then go through a certain number of basic routines followed by a brief abs and cool-down finale. The music is changed every few months to keep it fresh

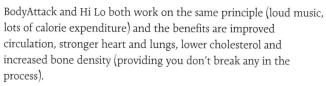

Here's an idea for you

If your gym does a class called Cardio Low or Cardio Jam you may want to try that as a gentle introduction to Hi Lo. If not, then find the instructor and explain your choreographic limitations – he'll tell you which of the weekly classes tends to be the most hardcore. If your gym does both, then BodyAttack is an easier place to start out than some of the Hi Lo classes.

but the exercises remain the same. There's a mix of work on the spot, forward–backward advances and movements circling the studio. A huge amount of hopping is involved, not recommended for those with joint problems or weak shins. Good cross-trainers are essential.

Hi Lo is very much open for interpretation and will vary wildly from one gym to the next and one instructor to another. A normal programme would kick off with 5–10 minutes of warm-up, then a peak of 20–30 minutes of target heart range dancing, followed by 20 minutes of body sculpting (a muscle-stretching floor session) and ending with cool-down and stretches. The Hi Lo refers to the mix of high and low intensity moves which is a coded warning that the class may get a bit frenetic (lots of leaping). It also usually means that there will be some challenging choreography with the instructors allowed to get creative. Classes will be a lot more fun for regulars, but can be off-putting for others unless they're particularly good at picking up new moves.

48. Vicious circuits

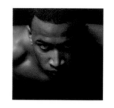

A complete body workout in the space of a single lunch hour? That, in a nutshell, is the appeal of circuit training.

Circuits are a great way to pack in a lot of variety and hard work in a short period of time. Variety, because a circuit can consist of a dozen or more different exercises which mix and match strength and cardio workouts, and hard work because knowing you only have a couple of minutes on each makes it easier to go for it. A well-organised circuit alternates between strength and cardio stations, or between upper and lower body so that each station functions as an 'active rest' period for the last. Since stations change according to the whim of the instructors you may also find yourself trying exercises you wouldn't normally do.

Here's an idea for you

At first you'll probably find circuit training sessions quite enough to leave you exhausted, but as you get better you may want to make individual stations more demanding. For press-ups, try putting your feet (or shins if that's too tough) up on a bench, or rest one foot on the heel of the other to focus a little more on balance. For crunches, try to perform the crunch while also keeping both legs off the ground to work the lower abs a little.

Typical moves included in a circuit are squats and step-ups (using a bench) to work the lower body, plus crunches and bicycle kicks for the abs. Favourites include press-ups to work the chest and some explosive work such as jumping jacks (star jumps). Shuttle runs and skipping are commonly included to keep the heart rate up and add an endurance factor to the circuit. The usual rule of thumb is that circuit training is about *compound* exercises that work as many muscles as possible at once. Where there are weights they will be light and the aim is to do as many repetitions as you can manage during the session. Session lengths may vary but 60 seconds is common and the overall goal is maximum fitness result in minimum time – something we can all relate to.

49. Squat yet bijou

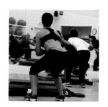

Squats power up your thighs, hips, calves and buttocks, and using free weights they also work your back, abs and obliques. It seems a shame to leave them to powerlifters.

Squats train your body in balance, they strengthen the stabilisers and tone the thighs and buttocks. They can increase flexibility and range of movement, they provide the driving force for runners and jumpers, and with attention to form they can protect your back from the wear and tear of daily life. Yet most of us shy away from them.

The basic squat can be done with nothing more than your own bodyweight if you prefer, and adding a barbell should be done when you're ready. Small weights and good form will do far more for you than large weights hefted around with scant consideration for your back.

Here's an idea for you

Try one-legged squats. Start off with legs slightly bent, shoulder-width apart and with a single dumbbell held in both hands on the top of your chest. Lift your right foot up so your calf is parallel to the floor. Bend your left leg at the knee and slowly lower your body. If you can make it to the point where your thigh is parallel to the floor, bravo; if not, stop before. Smoothly straighten your leg to return to the starting position.

119

Start off with your feet shoulder-width apart and your legs very slightly bent at the knee. Breathe in and pull your shoulders back a little so that your spine assumes its natural curve in your lower back. You may find it more comfortable to open the stance slightly by pointing your toes outwards. Just remember that your knees must move in the same axis as your feet, so toes outwards means your knees move outwards too – otherwise you'll set up a turning force and risk strain.

With your arms out straight in front, bend your knees and ease yourself down as if sitting into an armchair. The lift is done by straightening those knees and driving down through the legs and heels. If you find yourself lifting onto the balls of your feet, then you are unbalanced forwards. Keep the whole sole of your foot firmly on the floor.

50. Ab attack

Fab abs are top of the wish list for men and women alike. So why do so many people just stick to the basic crunch and hope for the best?

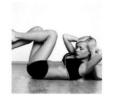

Stomach muscles don't have the ability to bulk up like other muscles so don't worry about working them too hard. You can work them too often though – light abs work can be done daily but after a hard session they need a day off just like any other part of your body if they are to repair damage and grow stronger. Remember that it's while you rest that you get stronger. Good exercises to focus on if you only have a few minutes to spare for the mat are twisting oblique raises and bicycling. These together hit pretty much the whole midsection.

For twisting oblique raises, adopt the normal crunch position on your back with legs bent. Now drop both knees to one side and

Here's an idea for you

The key to tone is tautness, and the key to tautness is keeping those abs contracted throughout exercises, and indeed throughout the day. One approach is to tie a piece of string around your waist (under your clothes of course) so that if you let your belly out it will touch the string. Whenever your tum touches the string you pull it in, effectively exercising your abs all day long.

keep them there as you lift the shoulders off the floor. Don't come up too high. After about 30 degrees your hip flexors take up the movement and the effort on your abs and obliques is reduced. Take it nice and slow.

For bicycling, start on your back with your legs straight and raise them both a few inches off the ground. Don't rest either leg back on the ground for the duration of the exercise. With hands on ears, lift your shoulders off the ground in classic crunch style. You should bend your left knee and bring it up towards your chest, simultaneously twisting so your right elbow reaches down to meet it. Alternate elbows/knees and keep the whole movement as slow and smooth as you can.

51. Cable manners

Cable stations aren't just something you find on skiing holidays. Cable and pulley systems offer the safety of machines with the flexibility of free weights.

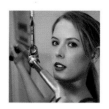

Cable stations consist of a stack of weights hooked up to a handle by means of a cable which runs over a pulley. Legions of strength trainers absolutely swear by them. Cable/pulley weights give you a lot of freedom of movement which lets you work muscles differently. Cable weights also apply pressure evenly throughout, which makes your muscles work through their entire range of movement. In a lot of free weights moves there is a point where balance means that your muscle is actually resting – such as the top point of a curl before your arm starts lowering again. With a cable, however, the thing is always pulling against you for as long as you have it in your hand. With that in mind, here are a couple of exercises to try.

Here's an idea for you

One of the handle types you may see lying around near the base of the station is a rope handle. Try this for pull down/up exercises and you'll find that it makes them much harder because it is more difficult to grip and so works the forearm and wrist muscles.

Cable crossovers

You'll need a crossover station here, with a set of weights/pulley/cable on each side of you. Set the cable to a low pulley on each side and with a handle in each hand start with your arms out away from your sides. Now bring your hands together until your wrists cross in front of your face, then slowly return to the starting position. That works shoulders and pecs.

Seated triceps extension

Pull a bench over to the low pulley and sit down with your back to the machine. Hold the bar in both hands and pull up so that your arms are straight up above your head. Without moving your upper arms, bend your elbows so your forearms go back and your hands end up behind your head with your forearms parallel to the floor. Straighten your arms again.

52. Progress report

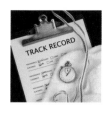

If you don't know what you're trying to achieve, how will you know if you've done it? Let's look at some ways to monitor progress.

Without a clear sense of progress it's easy to lose motivation, and vague goals make it hard to measure solid achievements. So here are a few ideas for measuring your own progress.

Weight

Chances are that you don't really want to lose weight; what you want to lose is fat. Muscle is denser than fat so it is entirely possible that exercise will successfully swap fat for muscle but leave your weight unchanged. Stop thinking weight and start thinking about how much of that weight is fat, and measure your body fat percentage. The easiest way is to use an electric body fat monitor. These pass a tiny electrical current through your body. Fat, muscle

Here's an idea for you

Find your BMI yourself. Take your height in metres and multiply the figure by itself. Then take your weight in kilograms and divide the weight by the height squared. Or you could look it up – there are plenty of BMI calculators online.

and water all conduct electricity at different speeds and so, given a bit of information about your height, weight, age and sex, the monitor can produce a figure for your body fat percentage.

Another figure that's often used is body mass index, or BMI, the relationship of your weight to your height. It's doesn't take into account your build or muscle mass, but it's a better guide to your shape than weight alone.

Strength

Do as many press-ups as you can in one go. If you're male, under 30 and you can do 45 or more, great; 35–44 is average. If you're 30–40, then over 35 press-ups is impressive, 25–34, average. Between 40–50, 30 or more for tough guys, 20–29 for average Joes. For women (using knees on the ground press-ups) under 30, 34 press ups or more for the superfit, 17–33 for the average. Aged 30–40? Then 25 means you're superfit; 12–24 and you're average. Between 40–50, those who can do 20 or more are the fittest; those capable of 8–19 are fine.

brilliant ideas

This book is published by Infinite Ideas, creators of the acclaimed **52 Brilliant Ideas** series. If you found this book helpful, there are other titles in the **Brilliant Little Ideas** series which you may also find of interest.

- **Be incredibly creative**
- **Catwalk looks**
- **Drop a dress size**
- **Enjoy great sleep**
- **Find your dream job**
- **Get fit!**
- **Heal your troubled mind**
- **Healthy children's lunches**
- **Incredible sex**
- **Make your money work**
- **Perfect romance**
- **Raising young children**
- **Relax**
- **Seduce anyone**
- **Shape up your bum**
- **Shape up your life**

For more detailed information on these books and others published by Infinite Ideas please visit www.infideas.com.

See reverse for order form.

Qty	Title	RRP
	Be incredibly creative	£5.99
	Catwalk looks	£5.99
	Drop a dress size	£5.99
	Enjoy great sleep	£5.99
	Find your dream job	£5.99
	Get fit!	£5.99
	Heal your troubled mind	£5.99
	Healthy children's lunches	£5.99
	Incredible sex	£5.99
	Make your money work	£5.99
	Perfect romance	£5.99
	Raising young children	£5.99
	Relax	£5.99
	Seduce anyone	£5.99
	Shape up your bum	£5.99
	Shape up your life	£5.99

Add £2.49 postage per delivery address

Final TOTAL

Name: ....

Delivery address: ....

....

....

E-mail:...............................Tel (in case of problems):

By post Fill in all relevant details, cut out or copy this page and send along with a cheque made payable to Infinite Ideas. Send to: Brilliant Little Ideas, Infinite Ideas, 36 St Giles, Oxford OX1 3LD. **Credit card orders over the telephone** Call +44 (0) 1865 514 888. Lines are open 9am to 5pm Monday to Friday.

Please note that no payment will be processed until your order has been dispatched. Goods are dispatched through Royal Mail within 14 working days, when in stock. We never forward personal details on to third parties or bombard you with junk mail. The prices quoted are for UK and RoI residents only. If you are outside these areas please contact us for postage and packing rates. Any questions or comments please contact us on 01865 514 888 or email info@infideas.com.